Stressed Out?

Causes, Effects, Solutions

Luis M. Rodriguez
Website: www.ahappybetterlife.com
Email: LMRod@ahappybetterlife.com

Disclaimer

The content of this book is intended for general information purposes only and not as a substitute for individual therapy as all of the advice may not be right for you. This book is not intended as a substitute for the medical advice of physicians. The reader should regularly consult a physician in matters relating to his/her health and particularly with respect to any symptoms that may require diagnosis or medical attention. Before beginning any new exercise program, it is recommended that you seek medical advice from your personal physician.

The publisher and author are not responsible for any specific health or allergy needs that may require medical supervision and are not liable for any damages or negative consequences from any treatment, action, application, or preparation to any person reading or following the information in this book.

Table of Contents

Introduction

Stress is everywhere. You can find it in the various tasks and chores that you carry out whether it's at home or at your job. While everyone is familiar with stress, not many are able to explain what it actually is. So what is stress? According to the Mayo Clinic, *"stress is a physical, mental, and emotional response to a challenging event and not the event itself"*. Stress responses occur when you feel threatened by something either real or imagined. Moreover, because of this you may panic or find yourself easily agitated by trivial matters. If you constantly feel stressed and distressed then it is definitely time for you to learn how to manage your stress levels so as to prevent it from taking a toll on your wellbeing.

Of course, stress doesn't necessarily have to be bad, in fact, whether it's positive or negative it is a normal part of everyday life. Having appropriate amounts of stress can actually be a good source of motivation as it can drive you to strive harder to achieve your goals. Negative stress however can diminish your quality of life affecting you both mentally and physically.

There are numerous ways of managing stress with there not being an absolute right or wrong way to deal with stress. If you try one way to manage your stress and it doesn't work for you don't let that stop you. Instead, try different methods until you find one that is best for you.

Stress and You

Everyone knows that stress exists. You deal with it every single day of your life. Every minute of each day you may be experiencing different levels of stress without even noticing it. However, what you may not understand is how stress affects you. It can change who you are, what you think, and how you feel. However when it rises above a threshold level, you will start to feel the anxiety rising in you. You may also be easily agitated or feel fatigued due to the stress you are experiencing.

As humans, we all cope with stress in our own way. Some may choose to ignore it, which really isn't coping, and that can lead to more serious physical and mental health issues. Others just allow themselves to be beaten down by it, which can be even worse. Whichever way you choose to deal with stress the fact remains the same: Stress does affect you and it shouldn't be ignored.

If you do choose to ignore stress, your body will begin to feel overwhelmed. It's not healthy to let stress linger because holding in the things that are bothering you could lead to serious health risks. Most of us like to think we're strong and can handle anything placed in front of us. So what if you can run yourself ragged twenty-four hours a day? So what if you can muster up energy on only two hours of sleep?

No prizes are given out for that type of lifestyle and none of these things will matter when stress decides to blow up in your face. So just how does stress affect a person?

If you don't take the time to defuse the stressors you're facing you'll soon find you can't think as clearly and you may even become filled with rage. Furthermore, your body can only take so much abuse. When your body and mind have been filled with enough pain and aggravation, you begin to weaken without even realizing it. And the effects of this weakening process will change who you are and why you exist. You'll also start to notice changes for the worse in your physical health.

Stress poses some significant health risks such as high blood pressure, heart disease, diabetes, and gastric problems. It can lead to weight gain, premature aging, and simply feeling more aches and pains. It can also cause you to become irritable, agitated, exhausted, hopeless, defiant, submissive, and antisocial.

Choosing to run from stress will not stop it. Stress can and will catch up to you no matter where you flee or where you try to hide. Instead face the challenge head on, don't let it beat you down so badly that the person you once were is lost.

Conversely, you can use stress to your advantage by learning how to process stress in a positive way. You can learn to cope with it effectively and to channel it so you don't let the little things wear you down. Just take the time to think about the situation confronting you then you decide how you can use it to move forward. Harness the energy normally wasted on stress and use it to fuel your ambitions. Don't be afraid of stress; instead control it so that you use it in a positive way.

How stress affects a person varies from person to person but it doesn't have to alter your personality. It doesn't have to be a demon and it doesn't have to cause chaos in your life or in the lives those you love. You can manage it and you can be the winner in stressful situations.

Identifying Stress and It's Effects

In order to fight stress and decrease stress levels in your life you must first identify it and make sure you know your plan to overcome stress, including short terms targets and long-term goals.

The fight or flight theory comes into play when you're faced with increasing stress giving you two ways to address the problem. The first is to distance yourself from the situation thus solving the immediate need for stress relief (but not necessarily solving the problem). The second is dealing with the problem, solving or eliminating it and simply fighting the stress away. These are the two options you have when dealing with increasing stress and in many cases, it is recommended you stay and fight. Although there may be situations where the best option is to simply get away from the stressful situation.

One example where getting away from the situation may be your best option is a failing marriage. The constant day after day fighting, arguments and insults inevitably creates an ongoing stressful life. While most people's first instinct is to run from the situation right away, most choose to stay and fight. Only after all attempts to solve the problems and trying to salvage the relationship fail do they choose to end the marriage.

People forget that they have the option of distancing themselves from the situation. They are determined to solve a potentially unsolvable problem sometimes leading to years and years of constant stress and the inability to advance.

Almost everyone suffers from stress at some point in his or her lives and you are no exception. Stress has real and clear physical symptoms; it is not confined strictly to your head. There are many physical symptoms that accompany increased stress. If you think about it for a minute, you will understand that it is very easy to spot a stressed out person when you see one.

Stress may cause sleep problems including a lack of sleep, the inability to sleep or oversleeping, which are all potential indicators of stress. Back or neck pain and stiffness are indications of stress as well as some headaches.

The digestion system also suffers the effects of stress including heartburn, gas, stomach pain, cramps, constipation, and diarrhea. Hair loss has been found to be related to increased stress levels. Skin problems may also be stress related and in some cases causing the problems and in others making them worst. Conditions such as psoriasis and eczema tend to become significantly worse under stress.

Everyone reacts differently to stress, some people get into a semi depressive mood and stop eating and lose weight, while with others it can have the opposite effect. Stress is also a main reason for chronic fatigue.

Stress is one of the main causes of heart disease and heart attacks as it has a strong connection with all of the symptoms such as heart pain, high blood pressure, palpitations or irregular heartbeat, pain in the chest, pressure on the chest, inability to breathe, sweaty palms and cold or hot flashes.

On the emotional side, stress has even clearer symptoms. It is surprising to find that people ignore these emotional warning signals or get used to them without questioning the reasons behind them. If you feel that you are experiencing a few of these symptoms you might be suffering from increasing stress. It is not difficult to identify signs of emotional stress which include an increased sense of nervousness or anxiety, symptoms of depression (moods swings, anti-social feelings), an edgy feeling, anger and frustration, lack of concentration, memory problems and a tendency to over react to situations.

What Causes Stress?

If you knew the leading causes of stress in your life, would you take action to eradicate them? Can you eradicate stress or is it an inoperable condition that will be with you all of your life possibly causing your eventual death? While there are many causes of stress, the following are some of the more common examples. Which one is your leading cause of stress?

1. Finances

Most studies agree that finances are a leading cause of stress. In 2005, Life Care, Inc. conducted an online poll in which 23 percent of the respondents named finances as the leading cause of stress in their lives. Financial stress has led the list in many modern polls.

People who said that finances was the leading cause of stress cited major purchases they have to make, such as a buying home or car while others are stressed by a loss of income or mounting credit card debt and the fear of bankruptcy. College students stress over paying for an education, Baby Boomers and older senior citizens find that the fear of not having sufficient income for retirement can be a major cause of stress.

2. Work

Work as a stressor was a close second as one of the leading causes of stress in that same Life Care, Inc. poll. 21 percent of respondents said it was the main reason for their stress. Our jobs or careers seem to be a cause of constant stress but how is it that the workplace a cause of stress?

Sometimes work stress is brought on by others, sometimes we bring it on ourselves. We worry about getting and keeping a job in order to provide for our families.

We worry about new types of work or new responsibilities and the constant struggle to climb a career ladder while being overwhelmed by the demands and pressures of the job. Changing work conditions or not getting along with coworkers or the boss can also place a strain on a person. Students, especially teenagers and college age students, cite schoolwork as a cause of stress.

3. Family

As wonderful as our families may be, they can still be a leading cause of stress. Whether it's an argument between you and your spouse or other family members, a divorce, a marriage, a child moving out, an aging parent moving in, the ebb and flow of family life is filled with stress.

Family health is also a leading cause of stress. A sick family member, a serious injury, pregnancy miscarriage or abortion all cause stress. Family changes of other kinds can bring stress as well Adoption, relocation and job changes for just one family member can cause stress for the entire family.

4. Personal Concerns

Personal concerns indirectly created by others are another top cause of stress with lack of control topping the list of personal concerns. We all have a deep-seated desire for control over our own lives. When that control is weak or missing in a given situation, we experience stress. For many of us a lack of control over our own time is a leading cause of stress. We want to decide when to do tasks around the home or at work. Holding a job, participating in the children's carpool to school, driving family to soccer practices, shopping, and scout meetings while trying to keep the household running can create major stress. You would like to control your life rather than let other demands control it but that is not always possible.

Being involved in legal proceedings can cause great stress as can wrestling with a bad habit or going through changes. Personal change of any kind can be a cause of stress.

5. Personal Health and Safety

Most people find that personal health is a leading cause of stress especially when the cause of that stress linked to obesity or a desire to lose weight. Other stressors can be personal bad habits that affect health and must be changed such as smoking, alcohol or drug abuse. Illness or injury, regardless of how serious, can be a leading cause of stress for many people. Personal health is more or less stressful according to the degree of seriousness and our personal outlook on health.

Personal safety is also a leading cause of stress. Women, more than men, tend to stress about their own and others safety. Adults tend to stress more than young people who may act invincible.

6. Personal Relationships

Whether it is friendship, dating, separation, marriage, divorce, or re-marriage, a relationship can be a leading cause of stress for many. We all want love and that is potentially available in relationships; but getting from A to B can be very stressful. Some resort to online relationships that are easier to handle while others withdraw and become reclusive. Either way the demands on time, finances, and emotions can cause ongoing stress.

7. Death

Probably the most wrenching cause of stress is the death of a loved one or close friend. Even the death of a pet can be stressful. Children are always a source of stress for parents but when a child dies, the stress is overwhelming. The same is true when a lifetime spouse passes on.

Win or Lose

Causes of stress change as we age. The stressed out child who threw tantrums becomes a young student being stressed by the school bully. The young student becomes a teenager, stressed by acne, hormones and dating. The teenager becomes a young adult trying to handle the stresses of leaving home, adjusting to college life, and managing finances. Life progresses to first jobs, marriage, children and so on.

Even if you move to a secluded cabin in the woods, stress will follow you.
Gaining knowledge of the leading causes of stress is important. Using that knowledge to win over unhealthy stress is vital.

Stress and Your Job

Stress at most jobs is unavoidable. It could be caused by a boss who is very demanding or a coworker who doesn't pull his or her weight. On the other hand, maybe you have a typically stressful position such as a doctor or lawyer. While some stress on the job can drive you to succeed and be healthy, too much can be bad for you. It can cause many problems and be detrimental to your health.

Because of this, it is important to learn some effective stress management techniques that you can do while at work. While many stress-inducing factors may be out of your control, like dealing with your boss, there are ways to cope that could save your life.

The average number of hours of work has gone up eight percent in one generation to 47 hours a week. One out of five Americans work as much as 49 hours a week. This can be a great source of stress not just at work but at home too. A high rate of divorces is credited each year to long hours at work.

It is important to realistically assess the hours you work each week. Can you cut back and still get the job done? Can you delegate your tasks to co-workers? Can you develop a more flexible schedule? If you consider these options, your job-related stress could diminish significantly.

Overworking can also cause a variety of health issues. You might become sick more often forcing you to either call in sick or show up for work sick, which is even worse. Work absenteeism is costing American companies a lot of money which makes workplaces less productive making you feel guilty for not showing up to work even if you are sick..

Americans also feel a great deal of stress because they no longer feel secure in their jobs. Continuing layoffs and company reorganizations provide little job security causing employees to live in constant fear that they will not have a job from one day to the next. This raises the concern of not having enough money in retirement funds for when it is needed. It is because of these factors that employees now have little loyalty to their employers, stress for both parties involved.

Since the workplace climate has changed, it is important that our own outlooks change as well. Employees need to reduce their stress even though they might not feel secure in their jobs. That might mean starting a part time business or opening a separate retirement fund and making regular contributions toward retirement. If you work on being proactive, chances are your stress levels will decrease. Face the fact that you are in charge of your destiny and take control of your future. You will feel a sense of freedom, and less unhealthy stress.

How to Manage Stress at Work

Regardless of what you have heard, stress plays a critical role in your life. It is a double-edged sword which can help you accomplish work in a timely and accurate manner, promote healthy competition and force you to evaluate problems and formulate creative solutions. It can also hamper your ability to effectively perform your job thereby reducing your chances of promotion, interfere with your capacity to sustain relationships and lead to physical illness. So how do you find a balance? You can start by preventing or eliminating unnecessary stress. Listed are seven ways to accomplish this.

1. Learn to manage your expectations. Are others clear about what you expect of them? Whether they are vendors, subordinates or peers, make sure they understand exactly what it is you're asking of them and when and how you would like it completed. This will prevent misunderstandings for you as well as the other person.

2. Effective communication. Many challenges arise due to a lack of or ineffective communication. Don't focus solely on your verbal and written communication though. Listening is a lost art for most people and one that can stand a little improvement. No matter what your position is, strong communication skills are essential.

3. Learn to let go. Are you someone who thinks that no one else can perform even the simplest of tasks as well as you can? If so, you could eliminate a lot of stress by simply learning to let go. Many companies reorganize departments into teams because they realize that it is a much more efficient and effective way to do business. It's not necessary for one person to perform all tasks related to his or her job. In fact, you are more effective when you concentrate on what you do best and let someone else take care of the rest.

4. Stop procrastinating. Staying on top of things and ensuring everything is flowing smoothly will reduce stress if the unexpected occurs. Procrastination often rears its ugly head when you are faced with a task you would rather not do. Instead of putting it off determine if it would be appropriate to delegate the project or a portion of it to someone else. If not get it out of the way first.

5. Schedule regular vacations. You are given vacation time for a reason. Some companies even require you to take time off. Being away from work gives you time to unwind, gain a new perspective, and become more focused. People who feel they are too important to the company and end up working too many hours without a break find themselves more prone to illness. When you become ill, it is your body telling you that you need to rest.

6. Address problems as they arise. Don't push issues to the back burner because you don't want to face them. Confront challenges as they arise in order to avoid becoming stressed from them building up and becoming seemingly insurmountable.

7. It is okay to say NO. Many people have difficulty saying no and then find themselves taking on every project, task, and role that is thrown their way. For projects outside your scope of responsibility, consider whether it will help you achieve your career goals and if not politely decline the offer and move on to something that will.

Ways Not To Deal with Stress

There are numerous stress management techniques for coping with stress in general and for dealing with both the physical and emotional causes of stress. There are also techniques for dealing with short-term symptoms of stress as well as long-term or chronic symptoms.

In your quest to deal with stress, you may also decide to attempt to deal with it on your own. While there are some do it yourself techniques that can be helpful, there are also some which can be counterproductive.

The following are some of the more counter-productive techniques.

In an attempt to alleviate the tension and worry that accompanies stress, you may head down a path where you will unwittingly engage in self-destructive behavior.

The type of stress that can lead to being short-tempered and cause you to behave angrily towards friends or family members can more often than not be heightened by excessive alcohol drinking or even coffee drinking which results in a high intake of caffeine. You probably won't see the connection between the cause and the symptom, which allows the cycle to continue causing even more stress than before.

Lack of sleep or insomnia is one of the most common causes of stress. Once again, the vicious cycle rears its ugly head. When something is troubling you and you are physically uncomfortable, it is difficult to relax enough to get to sleep. Moreover, when you don't get enough sleep you become fatigued and your tolerance level gets shorter. At this point, your ability to reason clearly becomes cloudy thereby causing the stress to continue. When you're in this type of a stress cycle even if you do manage to fall asleep, it's often an uneasy, interrupted sleep or not the type of deep sleep that is genuinely restful.

You may also try to cope with your stress by doing the right thing for the wrong reasons. One of the ways used to try and manage stress is focusing on something entirely different thereby taking your mind away from the stressful situation. However burying yourself in work or school projects as means of shifting your focus away from the problem may provide a change of focus but ultimately is not a productive way to deal with your stress. Avoiding your stress causing issues can at best be only partially successful and temporary.

Some problems do go away on their own and ignoring, or more accurately not over-reacting to them, can be a viable strategy. However, keep in mind that your problems and more importantly your stress will not disappear simply because you're not thinking about them.

Taking a step back to see things from a different perspective in order to get your emotions under control is healthy. Hiding your head in the sand is not.

Life is filled with obstacles that just seem to get in your way. The existence of those obstacles and the overwhelming need to overcome them when combined with doubts about your ability to do so leads to stress. Learning to evaluate and deal with life's challenges leads to the self-confidence needed to overcome and conquer your stress.

15 Practical Methods to Manage Your Stress

Taking an objective look at the circumstances and situations that seem unmanageable can be a helpful first step in dealing with stress. In addition, once you've identified the causes, having a plan in place to reduce the level of stress caused by each situation can be implemented.

Here are some practical methods to assist you in your effort to combat stress:

1. Be happy. Learn to laugh loud and hard. If you don't have a sense of humor, find someone else who does. Laughter releases endorphins, which are the happy chemicals, from the body and it helps boost your immune system.

2. Take control of your time and schedule. The most common cause of stress is not knowing what to do and feeling powerless about everything going on around you. You'll be better able to deal with stress if you have a good handle on your job, your relationships, and all your other activities. When you take control and empower yourself you are more inclined to stay focused and calm. Make a conscious decision that you are going to do

something about your problem instead of jus
thinking about it.

Remember to allow for the unexpected whethe
good or bad. Be flexible when it comes to
rearranging your schedule. Get up 15 minutes
earlier in the morning; thus allowing yoursel
adequate time to get to all your appointments

3. Avoid procrastinating on important or urgen
tasks. Whatever needs to get done, do i
immediately. Do any unpleasant tasks first so tha
you won't have to worry about them for the
remainder of the day. Keep track of your tasks and
check them off your list as you complete them
Don't rely on just your memory.

4. Focus your attention on the present moment
Whether it's the person speaking to you or the job a
hand, stay focused and you'll avoid making mistakes
so that it doesn't lead to more anxiety and tension.
If you have to wait for someone or something, be
patient. Anxiety caused by impatience raises your
blood pressure and leaves you vulnerable to more
serious illness. Say no to requests that you can'
accomplish and delegate trivial tasks. Remember
that you don't have to do everything. Break down a
job assignment into separate tasks and assign them
to people with the suitable skills.

5. Get out and exercise. Make exercise a habit by scheduling it into your daily routine. Do something you like such as walking, bicycling, swimming, or any activity that appeals to you. Exercising can considerably reduce your stress and while this won't solve your problem, it will lift some of the emotional intensity associated with your stress. Exercise also promotes the release of natural soothing chemicals, endorphins, in your body and you should begin to notice your sleep becoming more restful.

6. Find a support group. It's much easier coping with your stress if you have other people helping and supporting you. Studies have shown that married couples and people who are outgoing have considerably lower levels of stress in their lives.

When choosing the friends you hang out with be sure to choose friends who have a positive outlook and not ones who are worriers. The reason is that friends who continually put you down or have a negative attitude towards life will only add to your anxiety.

If you have a problem, invite a good friend to talk about your problem, it helps to just get it off your chest. Sometimes a long-distance call to an old pal can also be great therapy.

7. Learn to forgive instead of holding grudges. Don't expect others to be perfect and you won't be disappointed. Expect people to do the best that they can. Become more flexible and adaptable to your environment. Communicate clearly with your peers and boss. Ask questions and repeat instructions that you are given. Clarifying directions at the beginning of a project can save you a lot of time later on and helps to prevent misunderstandings. Be honest in your dealings with others. Lying and cheating leads to stress.

8. Practice breathing deeply and slowly. When we are stressed, we tend to tighten up and stop breathing. When you notice yourself doing that stop whatever you're doing and take several deep breaths; in through your nose and out through your mouth. Doing this calms your body and your mind. When you exhale, exhale slowly, and repeat the process several times. Focus on your breathing as it flows in and out. This is one of the best ways to relax in the midst of any activity. Following this practice allows you to find a breathing pattern that is natural and relaxing to you.

Make use of this yoga technique: Inhale slowly counting to four. Exhale through your mouth even more slowly counting to eight. Make a sighing sound as you exhale and feel the tension dissolve. Repeat this 10 times or for as long as you need,

9. Eat healthy. Try not to skip any meals especially breakfast, make time to eat heartily no matter how busy you may be. Take nutritious snacks to the office or anytime you're out and about. Keep in mind that a nutritionally balanced diet is essential to your health and lifestyle. Researchers have found that even small deficiencies of thiamin, a B-complex vitamin, can cause anxiety symptoms. Pantothenic acid, another B-complex vitamin, is critical during times of stress. Avoid caffeine, alcohol, and large amounts of sweets, which can only worsen your symptoms of stress.

10. Maintain a positive attitude. Be grateful for what you have especially when everything seems to go wrong. Make it a daily habit to write down all the things you appreciate and are grateful for in your life. Expressing appreciation for even the simplest things in your life will make a huge difference in the way you feel.

Don't exaggerate the complexity of your situation because every problem has a solution. All you need to do is find that solution. Learn to be happy and to enjoy life's blessings. You will become more resilient when you cultivate a positive attitude to situations in your life. Above all, live one day at a time.

11. Learn to accept things you can't change. Sometimes we stress over situations that are beyond our control and changing those difficult situations isn't always possible. When faced with such a situation learn to recognize this fact and accept it. In this way, you will be able to focus on the things you do have control over which you can change.

A classic situation is getting stressed and asking "why me". This only serves to exacerbate the situation. However, learning to ask empowering questions such as "what can I do to make this better" or "what can I learn from this" will ensure you don't stress over something you cannot control.

12. Enjoy life and all it has to offer. Allow yourself some time to enjoy simple pleasures to help ease your stress. Make an appointment to get a professional massage or trade massages with a loved one. Give yourself permission to enjoy a movie, watch a concert or sports event, listen to music, or read a book without feeling guilty about doing what you enjoy. Relax with a soothing cup of chamomile herb tea with a little bit of honey. Chamomile has long been used to relieve nervous tension.

Arrange a makeover day with a friend. Do each other's hair or paint your nails, chat, and laugh. You can make a simple steam facial at home with boiling water, adding aromatic herbs to the water for a sensual touch. Essentially pamper yourself!

13. Recharge your body and your mind. The main reason most stress occurrences are work related is because we spend a disproportionate part of our adult life at work. The more time you spend at work means less time spent on doing the things you love and enjoy doing. Schedule some private time for yourself every day, after all you deserve it. Setting aside this time and not allowing any intrusions means you are in a situation that you have created thus empowering you to make similar changes in other areas of your life. Silence your cellphone and enjoy a quiet evening alone or with your family. You may want to spend a few minutes writing your feelings out in a journal, which is beneficial in finding a different viewpoint in life, and helps relieve internal conflicts.

14. Practice meditation techniques. One of the simplest ways is to focus on your breathing, feeling your breathe fill your lungs and hearing the soft exhale. You can also repeat a word or phrase with an uplifting meaning while doing this. Get into the habit of doing this for 5 minutes gradually increasing the time to 20 minutes. Doing this daily helps to reduce high blood pressure and relieves other physiological responses to stress.

15. Schedule an activity that is a change in your usual routine. If your week is packed with scheduled meetings and assignments then on weekends, go out and do the opposite. Enjoy some relaxing and fun noncompetitive activities.

If you are struggling to finish work assignments during the week, use the weekend to work on a project that you can complete in a few hours. Take time out for a little entertainment in the middle of your workday. When the pressures of completing a project are too great, your productivity can drop. Take a walk or eat lunch outside the office.

Conclusion

While it is impossible to completely eliminate stress from your life, you can learn to manage it. Even though stress may sometimes be overwhelming, you should never let it run your life or stop you from accomplishing your goals. Instead, always take control of your thoughts and when necessary take a step back and re-evaluate the situation. If you are feeling stressed because you are afraid of making mistakes, take deep breathes to compose yourself. You should talk about your feelings with your friends and family because with the love and support from your loved ones, you will feel more confident to take on the world.